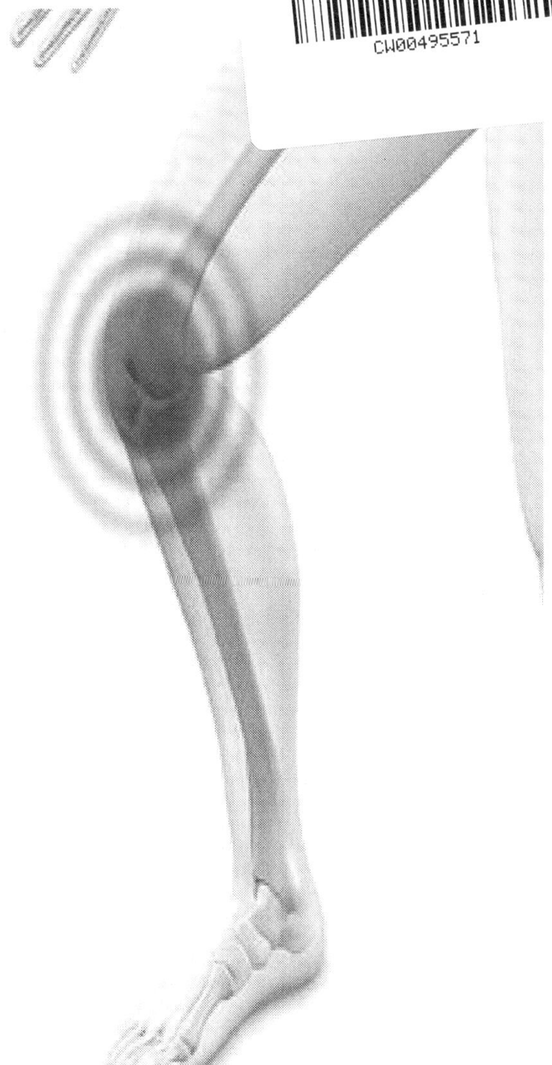

# BEST KNEE STRENGTHENING EXERCISES

Best Exercise to Relieve and prevent knee Pain, Rehabilitations, injuries and Replacements.

**CHARLINE GRIMMY**

# TABLE OF CONTENTS

# INTRODUCTION

Are you afraid of performing an exercise that you think it will worsen your knee pain or damage? The greatest thing you will like to do, as far as your doctor thinks it's OK, is to strengthen as well as improve the muscles that surround your knee. Begin gradually and start increasing your level of consistency. Consult your workout coach to determine which workout exercises are appropriate for you.

Knee discomfort can be a major hindrance in your day-to-day activities. It might be due to arthritis, tendinitis, traumas, or tight muscles. The good news is that you don't have to quit exercising because of it. Regular activity, regardless of the reason, is an excellent approach to cure and reduce knee discomfort.

The majority of these workouts are not too demanding. You may start reducing your knee pain right now if you make the appropriate actions.

In this book, we will discuss various workout exercises that will help you to strengthen your knee. What you need to know that these exercises are very effective and active to strengthen your muscles around your knee.

# PART 1: BASIC UNDERSTANDING AND BENEFITS OF KNEE EXERCISE.

People who suffer from knee arthritis may believe that workout is the last activity they will like to do but however, regular exercise on the other hand, can help most persons with knee osteoarthritis. In fact, studies show that regular exercise is just as beneficial as acetaminophen or nonsteroidal anti-inflammatory drugs (NSAIDs) in lowering knee arthritis pain.

Most knee exercise programs will reduce knee pain as well as enhance the muscles around the knee region. The advantages of knee exercises are discussed in this book, as well as specific stretching and strength training, including aerobic activities to get individuals started with.

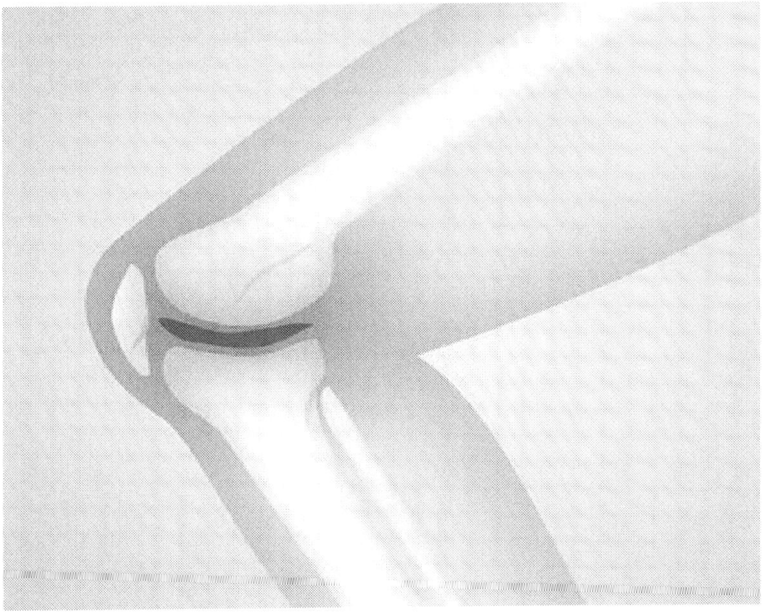

## BENEFIT OF KNEE EXERCISE

The followings are the benefits you will derive from knee strengthening exercises.

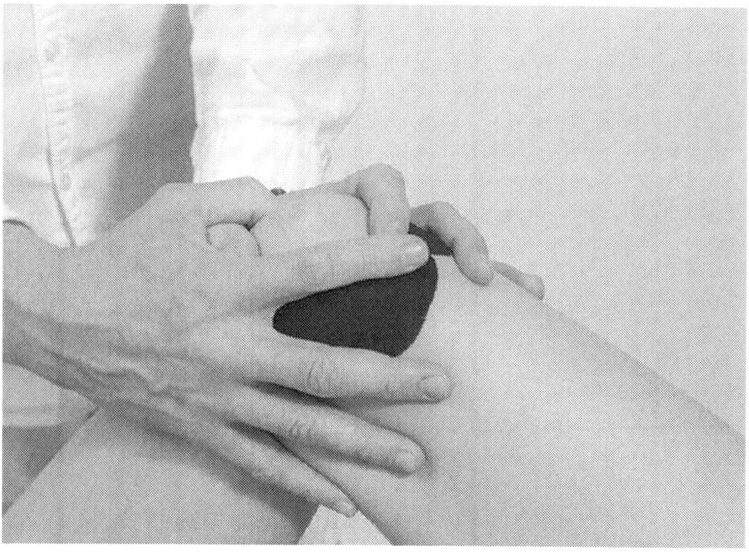

## IT HELPS TO ELIMINATE KNEE JOINT PAIN:

Muscles get healthier and stronger when you exercise regularly, and stronger muscles may continue to support joints. The knee is becoming more and more stable as well as bones suffer less pressure during joint movement as the quadriceps, hamstrings, including other muscles supporting the knee are strengthened, which lessens stiffness. Endorphins, the body's natural painkillers, are also released during exercise.

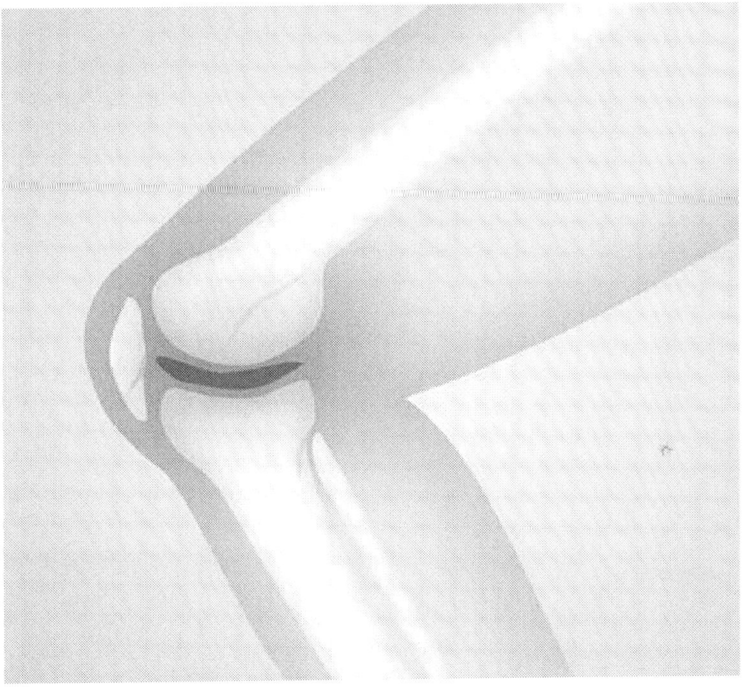

## KNEE FLEXIBILITY:

Pain can make a person less active, which may result in joint stiffness and muscular weakening, this can contribute to even greater pain. Regular physical exercises keep the knee joint as well as surrounding muscles flexible, which improves functional outcomes.

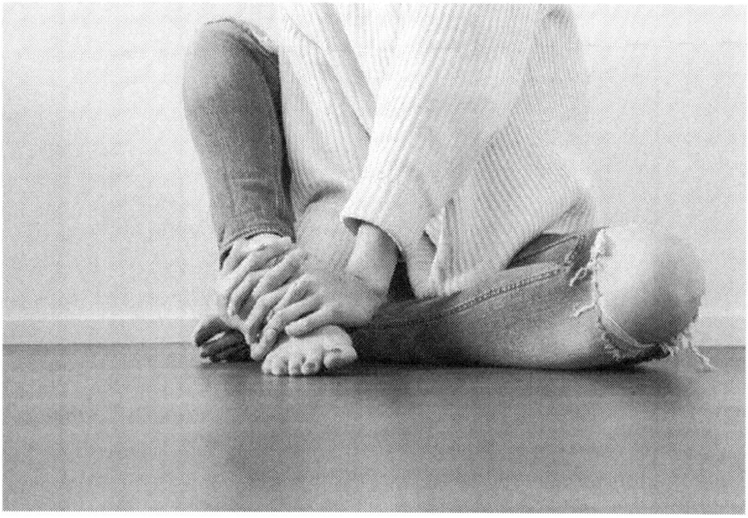

## REDUCES STIFFNESS:

Knee movement can increase by 20% with exercise —this implies that those who exercise regularly can observe real changes like bending their knees further, rising out of a chair more comfortably, as well as walking longer distances.

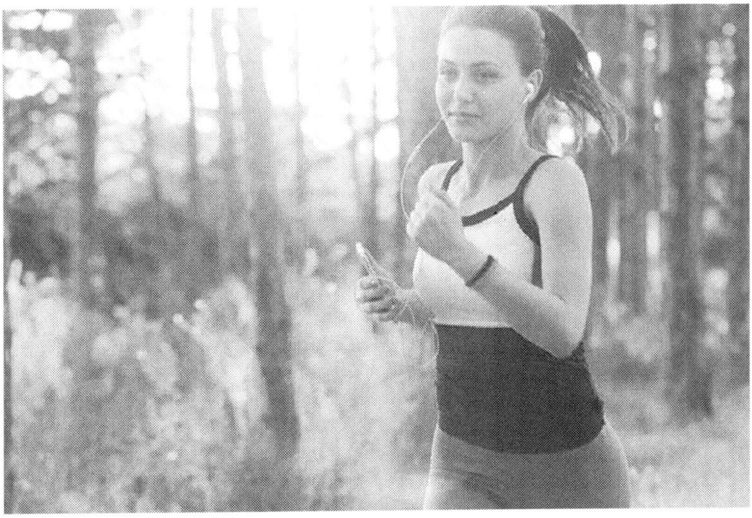

## KNEE JOINT CARTILAGE:

To keep healthy, joint cartilage requires mobility and a certain level of muscle mass stress. Synovial fluid is held in cartilage in the same way that water is kept in a sponge. The cartilage is pressed when the joint is utilized, and synovial fluid is produced, supplying nourishment and lubricant to the remainder of the joint.

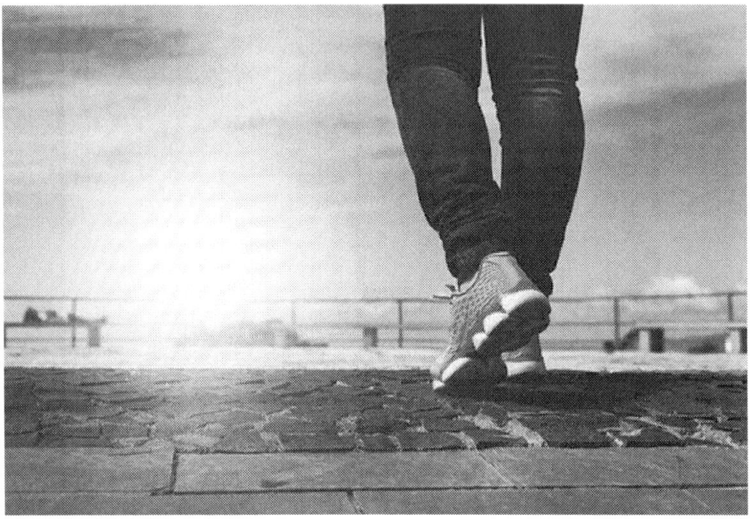

## REDUCES WEIGHT LOSS:

Workout combined with a plant-based diet, will help you lose weight and relieve stress on your knees. Weight loss has a multiplier effect.

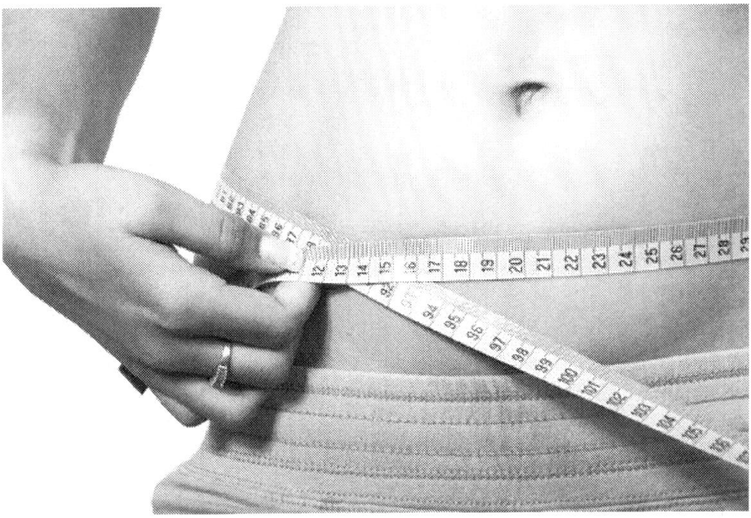

# PART 2: WARM-UP BEFORE KNEE EXERCISE

There is a need to do some post-workout exercises before you engage in knee exercises fully. This will boost your internal muscles and body reactions.

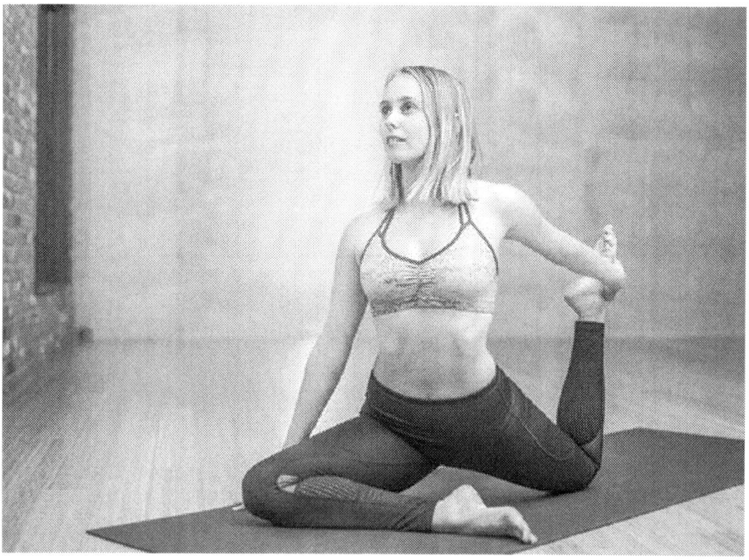

## POST-WARM UP:

A 10-minute warm-up routine should usually precede exercise. Warming up improves blood flow and physically activates the body, allowing muscles to become more flexible. A stroll or other slow-paced cardiovascular activity is a useful warm-up. A warm massage and modest range-of-motion exercises may be enough for individuals with severe arthritis.

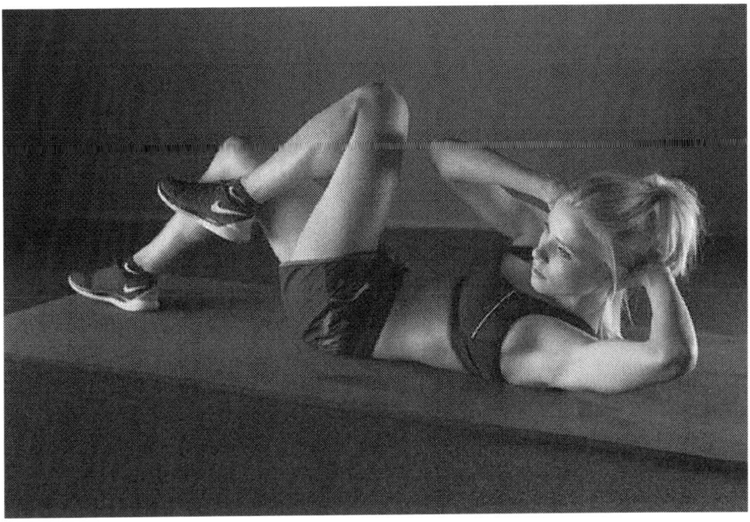

## POST LEVEL EXERCISE:

The knee may seem swollen as well as achy just after an exercise mostly for the first-timers who have not done knee exercise before, but there are things you can do to minimize swelling and ease discomfort. Some folks elevate their knees or apply a cold compress to their knees (a bag of frozen peas will do).

**NOTES:** If you experience continuous discomfort while performing knee exercise, stop and consult a healthcare expert or a competent sports trainer before proceeding.

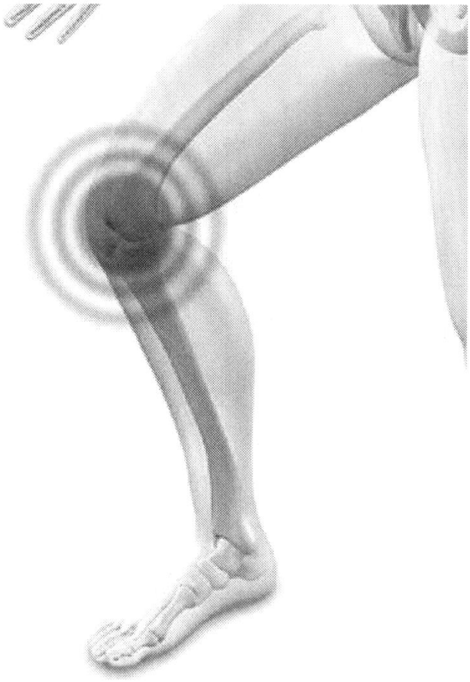

# PART 3: AEROBIC EXERCISE FOR KNEE ARTHRITIS

Aerobic workouts especially low basic impact aerobic fitness will assist most persons with knee arthritis.

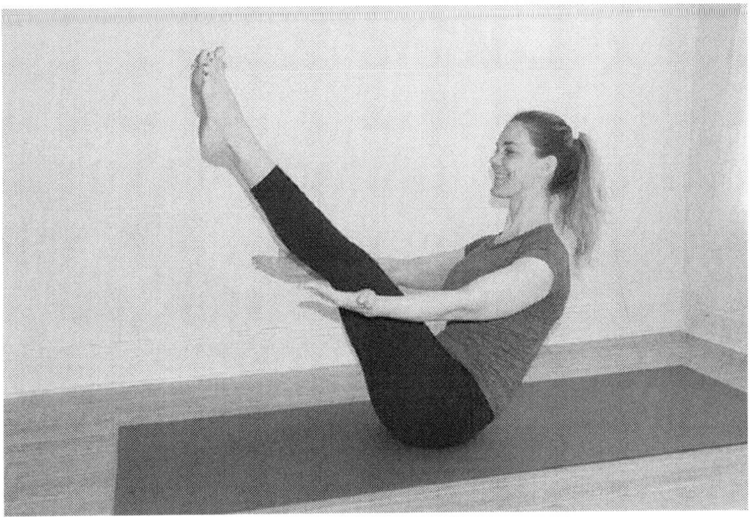

# AEROBIC EXERCISE THAT CAN STRENGTHEN YOUR KNEE

For those with minor or severe knee issues. The followings are aerobic exercises that can strengthen your knee joint including the muscles around the knee.

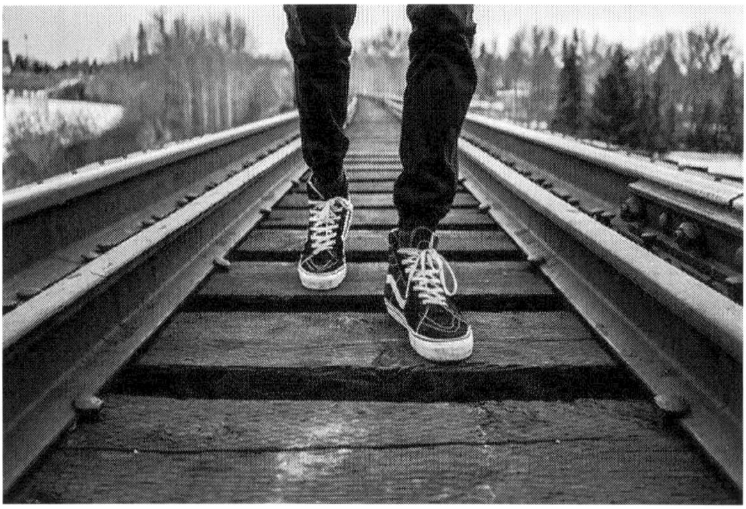

## WALKING:

For several people, walking is weight-bearing, yet nevertheless has little impact. It is possible to walk outside or on a treadmill. Persons suffering from knee arthritis cannot adapt the treadmill to an incline that might modify the mechanism of the body and put additional stress on the knee.

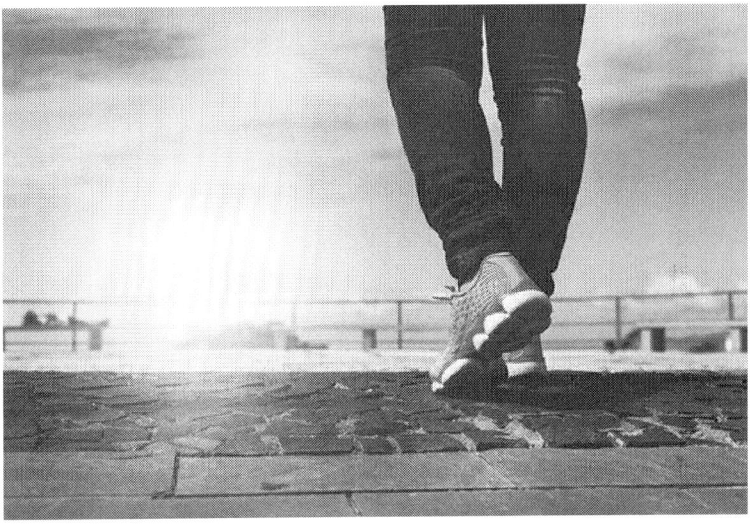

## CYCLING:

Cycling is another way that can strengthen the knee joint. When cycling you will notice pressure at the region of your knee. Cycling can also help to enhance the muscles around the knee.

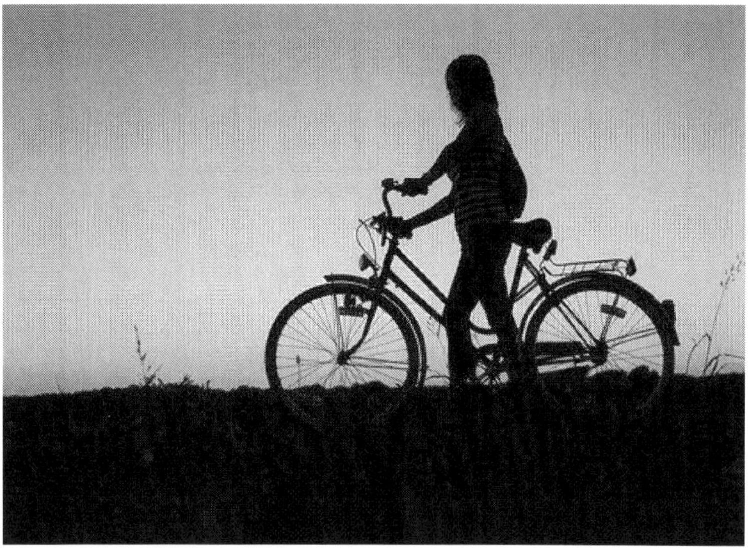

## SWIMMING:

Swimming is a wonderful way of aerobic exercise that is moderate on the knees and weighty joints. Swimming help to utilize pool water to avoid the likelihood of muscular strain; for instance, when swimming in a freestyle stroke, some people may have neck aches when not using adequate breathing methods.

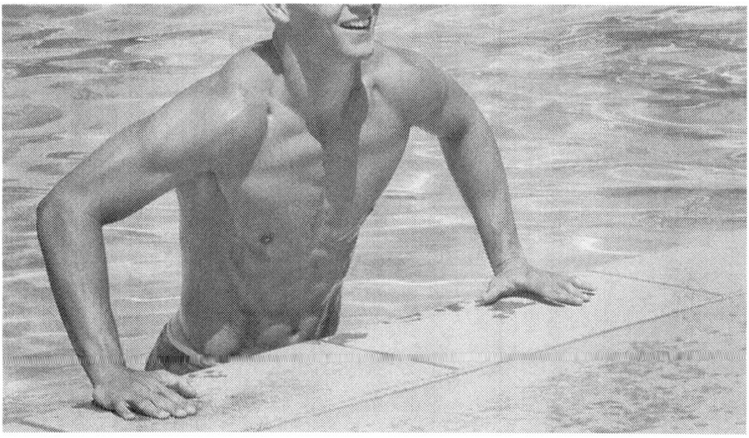

# PART 4: KNEE STRETCHING EXERCISE

Knee discomfort may throw a kink in your favorite hobbies, whether you are a competitive athlete, a weekend warrior, or a regular walker. Knee discomfort is a very prevalent problem. Based on the current Cleveland Clinic, 18 million Americans seek medical assistance each year for knee discomfort.

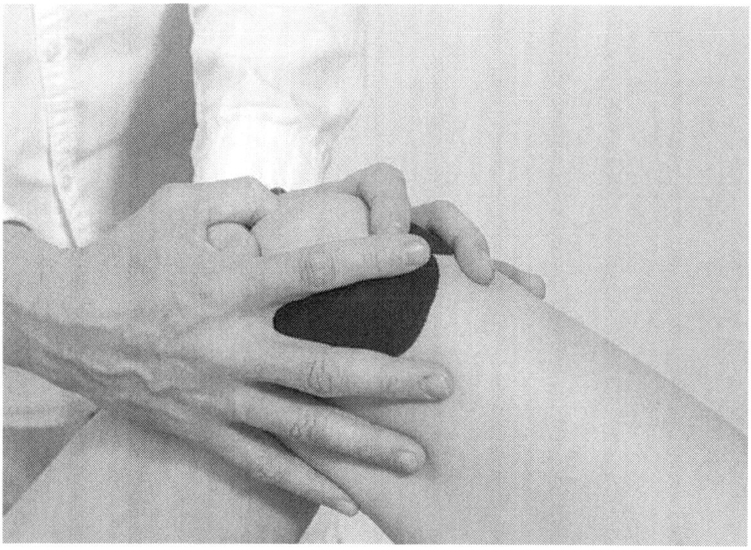

The excellent news is that knee discomfort may be treated in a variety of methods, including at-home stretch exercise as well as strengthening activities. We will lead you into some of the most intense workouts for strengthening your knee and reducing knee pain.

## IMPACT OF STRETCHING EXERCISE:

According to the Institute of Orthopaedic Surgeons, stretch exercise can assist enhance the range of movement as well as flexibility in your knee joint. This can help you move your knee more easily.

Warm-up for at least 5 to 10 minutes before beginning your stretching routine. Warming up with low-impact workouts like stationary cycling, walking, or utilizing an elliptical machine is an excellent idea.

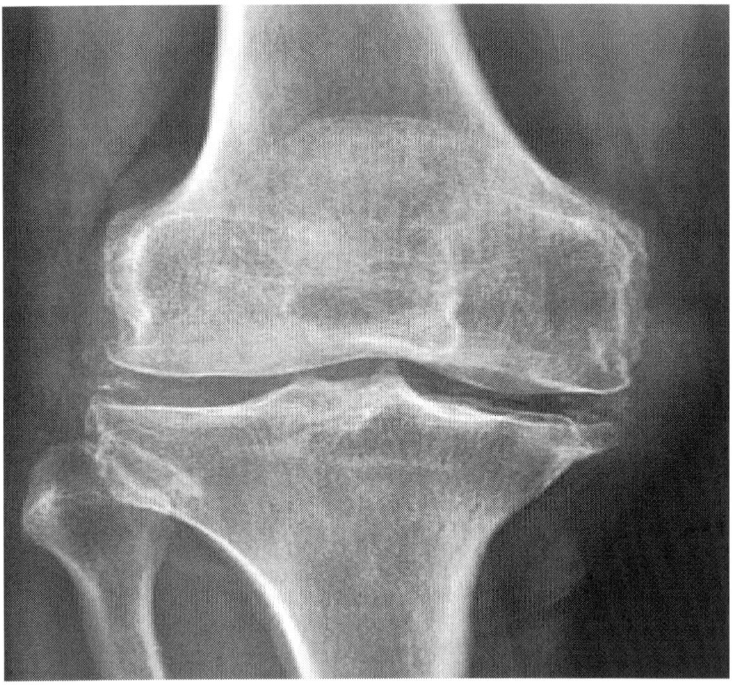

# BEST STRETCHING EXERCISE THAT WILL ENHANCE YOUR KNEE

The followings are stretching exercises that can enhance your knee joint and also the muscles around your knee.

## HEEL AND CALF STRETCH:

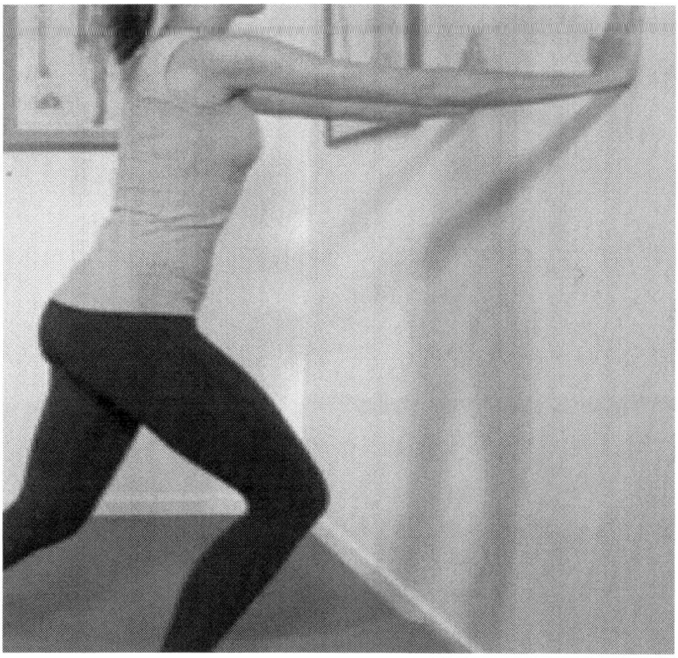

How to do this:

- Firstly, ensure that you stand straight.
- Your palm should be on the wall.
- Your feet should also be on the floor.
- The right leg should be forward while your left leg should be at the back.
- Maintain your posture.
- Lean forward with your knee and hold for at least 40 seconds.
- Repeat by changing the leg.
- Also, continue at least three times.

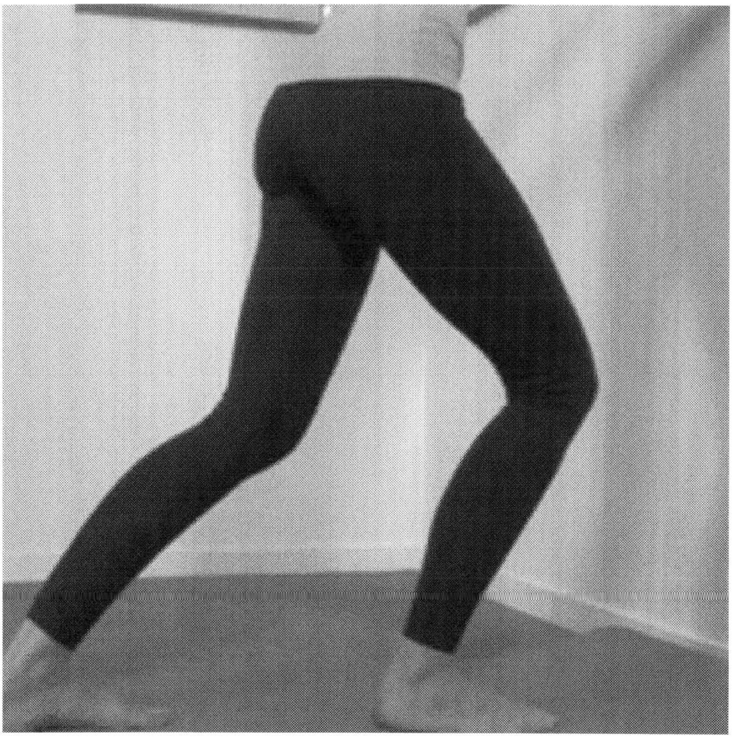

## KNEE-HOLD STRETCH:

- Firstly, lie strength on the floor.
- Your body position should be sideward on the floor.
- Maintain the position of your legs.
- Move your right hand backward and your leg bend in a backward direction.

- Hold your leg with your hand for at least 30 seconds to 50 seconds.
- Repeat the same with your left leg and hand.

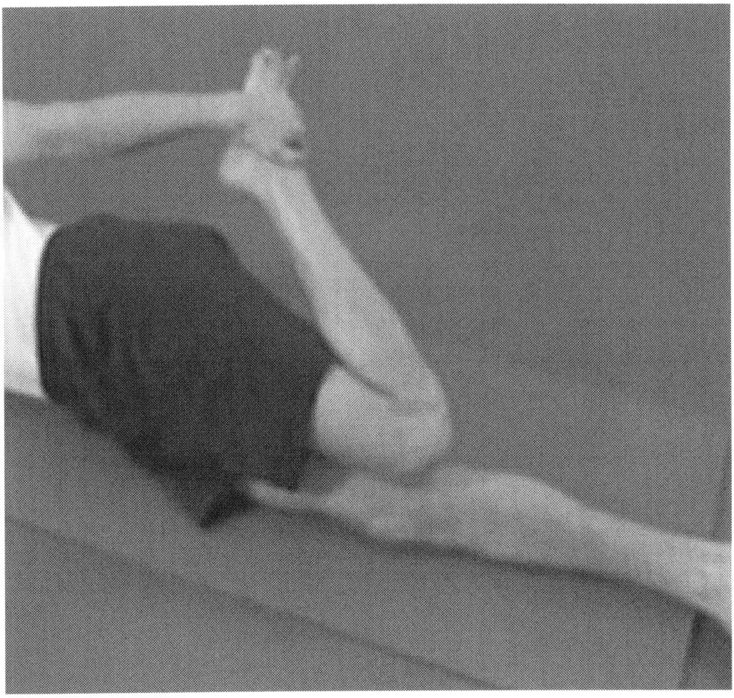

## QUADRICEPS STRETCH:

- Firstly, stand straight.
- Your feet should be on the floor.
- Pull your leg backward while your knee is bent.
- Move your hand backward to enable you to hold your foot.
- Ensure you hold for at least 40 seconds to 1 minute.
- Repeat the same with the other leg

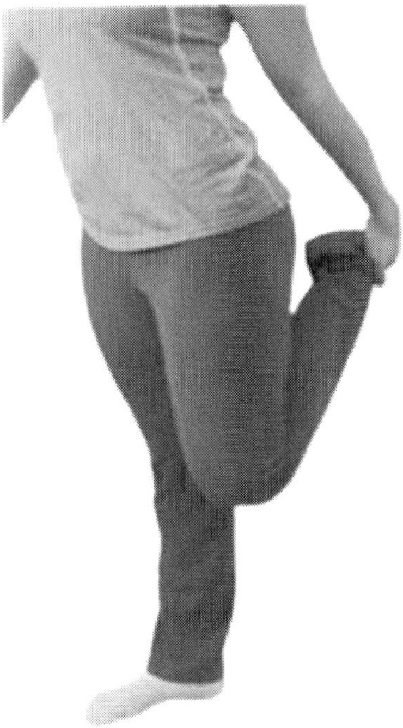

## HAMSTRING STRETCH:

- Lie flat on the floor.
- Your legs should remain straight.
- Raise your right leg upward.
- Hold your leg with your two hands while you move your leg a little bit forward and backward. Repeat the same with the other leg.

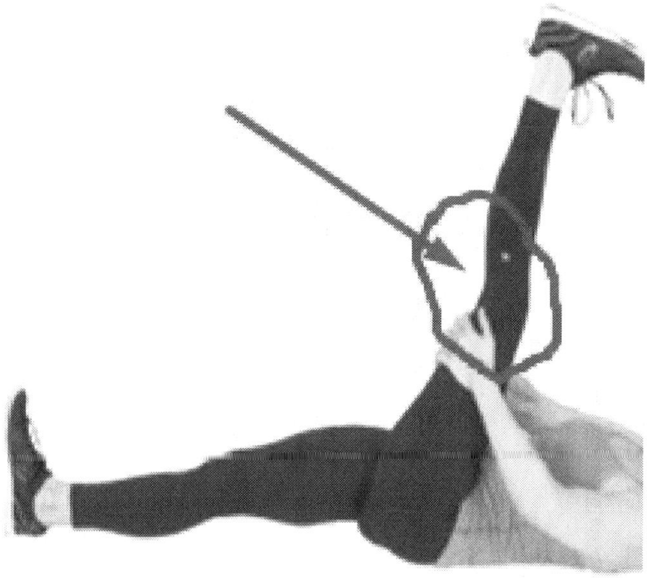

# KNEE STRENGTHENING EXERCISES

This can assist to relieve stress mostly on the region of your knee joint by regularly exercising the muscles that are around the knee region.

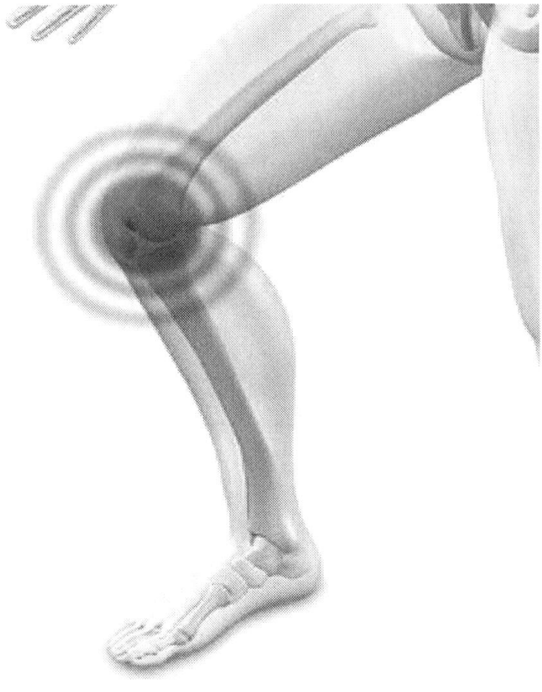

Focus on exercises your hamstrings, as well as quadriceps and glutes, also hip muscles to help strengthen your knees.

## HALF SQUAT:

Half squats are a great technique for your quadriceps as well as glutes and hamstrings to be stronger, without any tension. Get into a squat stance with the shoulder width of your feet apart. Put your hands on and out to straighten your hips.

Facing straight, approximately 10 inches squat gently. Stop for a few seconds, lift your heels then.

Make two to three sets with ten repeats.

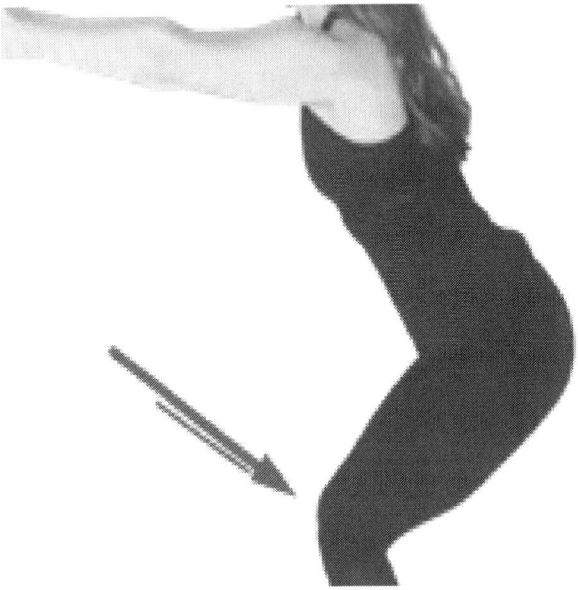

## CALF RAISES:

- Stand straight.
- Your legs on the floor.
- While your hands should on your waist.
- Lift your heel above the floor level.
- Gradually lower your heel downward, back to the initial position.
- Control is very essential so that you won't fall.
- Do 3 to 5 set 12 repetitions.

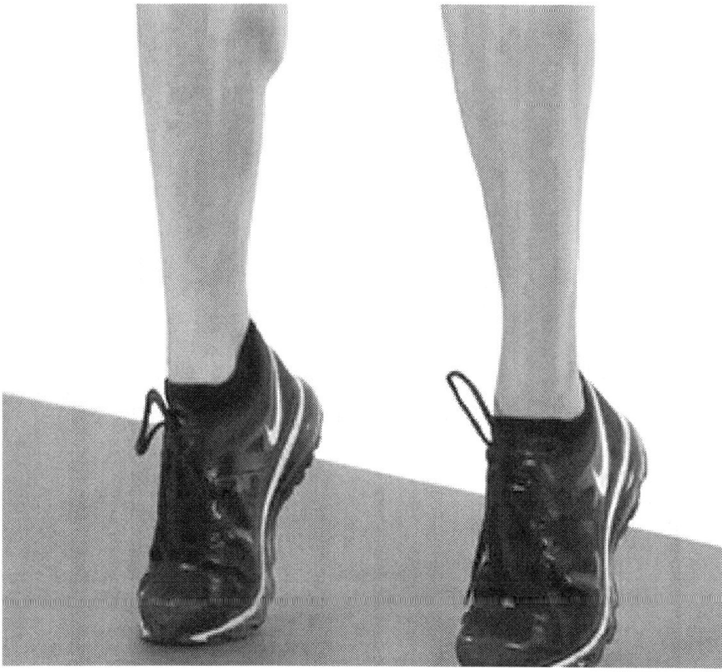

## LEG EXTENSIONS:

- Firstly sit on a chair.
- Your Foot should be on the floor while your knee is bent.
- Then look straight ahead, contract your thigh muscles as well as extend your right leg as high as possible without raising your buttocks from the chair.
- Do 2 to 3 sets and 12 reps for each leg.

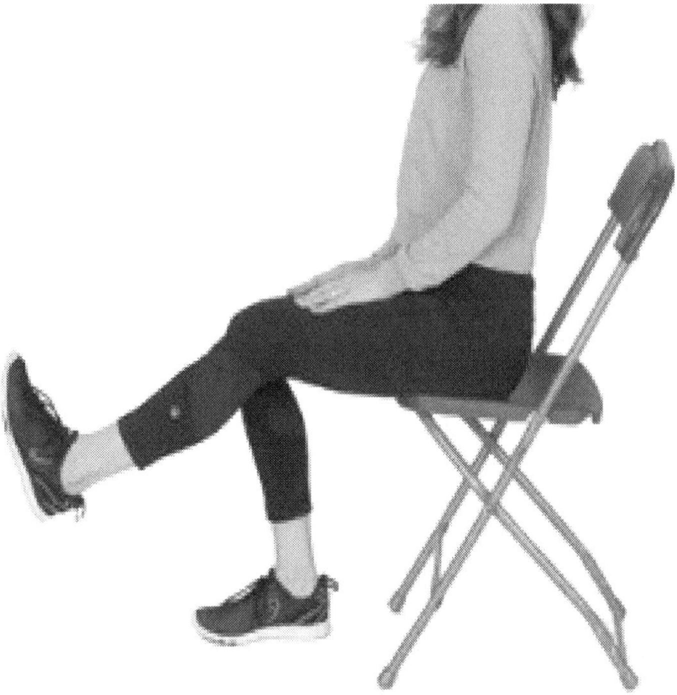

## STRAIGHT LEG RAISE:

The straight leg raise improves both your quadriceps and your hip flexion muscles. You should perhaps feel that your shins contract if your foot bends at the end of the action.

You may increase the weight of a 5-pound knee by increasing the weight of your legs to a higher degree.

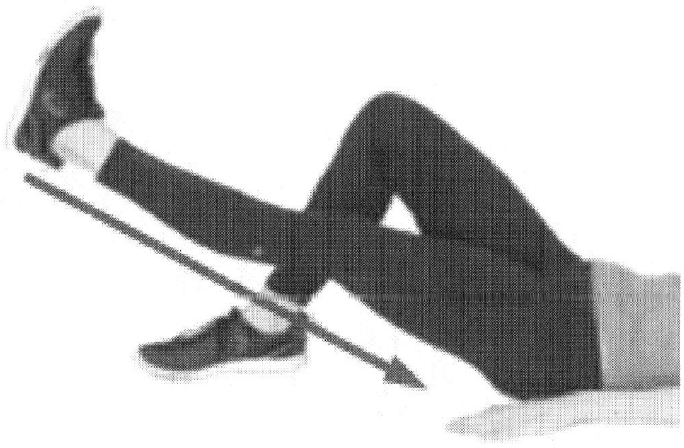

## SIDE LEG RAISE:

This workout strengthens both the muscles of your abductor's hip and your glutes. Your hip muscles, positioned outside your hips, will enable you to stand, walk as well as easily rotate your legs. It also Improving the muscles in the knees as well as ankles which will help to prevent and eliminate distress.

Side leg raise also put pressure on the knee region by that boost the knee muscles.

Since this workout is simple to do, you may bring a weight of 5 pounds to your knees and move gradually to a heavier level as your leg muscles acquire strength.

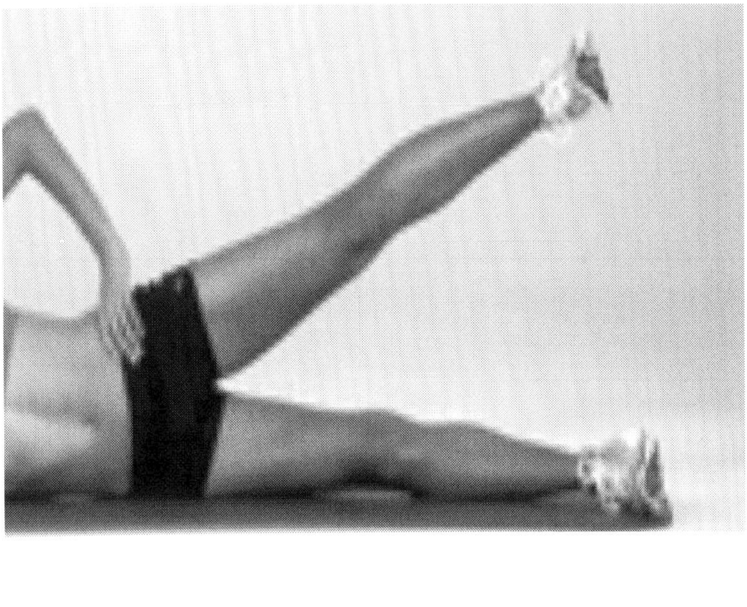

## PRONE LEG RAISE:

This workout targets both your glutes and your hamstrings. This exercise put more pressure on the knee. By that, it builds your leg muscles to a greater degree.

How to do this:

- Lie on the floor while your tummy and face facing towards the ground.
- Ensure that your legs are straight.
- Move your right leg upwards in your backward direction.
- Return to the normal position.
- Do it with your left leg.

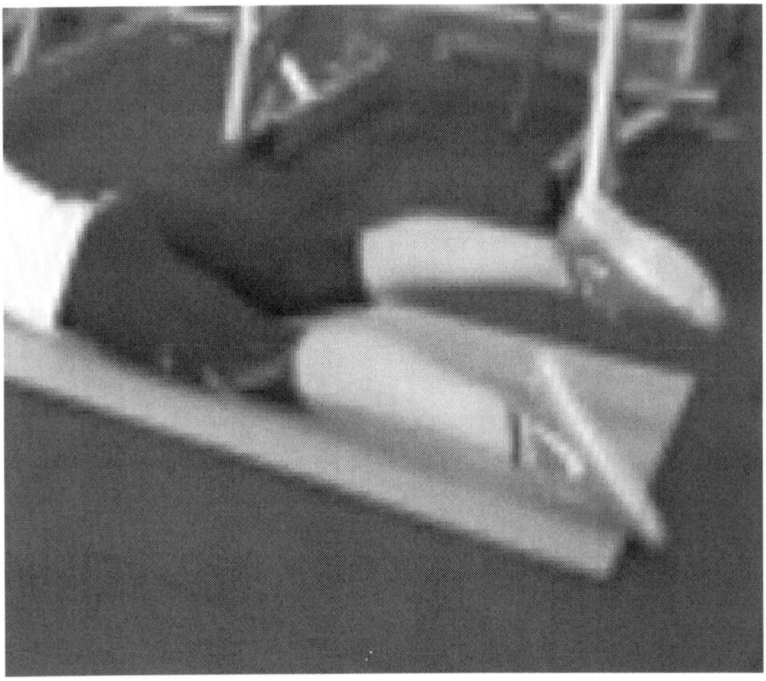

Printed in Great Britain
by Amazon

76174141R00026